Frequently Asked Questions

all about vitamin E

JACK CHALLEM & MELISSA DIANE SMITH

AVERY PUBLISHING GROUP
Garden City Park • New York

The information contained in this book is based upon the research and personal and professional experiences of the author. It is not intended as a substitute for consulting with your physician or other health care provider. Any attempt to diagnose and treat an illness should be done under the direction of a health care professional.

The publisher does not advocate the use of any particular health care protocol, but believes the information in this book should be available to the public. The publisher and author are not responsible for any adverse effects or consequences resulting from the use of any of the suggestions, preparations, or procedures discussed in this book. Should the reader have any questions concerning the appropriateness of any procedure or preparation mentioned, the author and the publisher strongly suggest consulting a professional health care advisor.

Series cover designer: Eric Macaluso
Cover image courtesy of Barry Axelrod Studios

ISBN: 0-89529-941-0

Copyright © 1999 by Jack Challem and Melissa Diane Smith

All rights reserved. No part of this publication may be reproduced, stored in a retrieval system, or transmitted, in any form or by any means, electronic, mechanical, photocopying, recording or otherwise, without the prior written permission of the copyright owner.

Printed in the United States of America

10   9   8   7   6   5   4   3   2

Contents

Introduction, 5

1. The Heart Protector, 9
2. The Cancer Preventer, 23
3. The Immunity Booster, 35
4. The Brain Preserver, 43
5. The Sexual Health Vitamin for Men and Women, 51
6. The Anti-Aging Nutrient and More, 57
7. Buying and Taking Your Vitamin E Supplement, 67

Conclusion, 79

Glossary, 81

References, 83

Suggested Readings, 87

Index, 89

Introduction

Could one single vitamin reduce your risk of developing heart disease, cancer, and Alzheimer's disease?

If the supplement is vitamin E, the answer is yes. Too incredible to be true? Just read a little further.

Discovered in 1922, vitamin E was for years the butt of jokes that referred to it disparagingly as the "sex vitamin" because its lack could cause sterility in rodents. Amazingly, as far back as the 1940s, Canadian physicians discovered that vitamin E could protect people from coronary heart disease. But because these doctors could not explain in scientific terms why vitamin E worked, they were dismissed as quacks and charlatans. For many years to come, vitamin E would be regarded as a "cure in search of a disease" and nothing more than a waste of money.

Fast-forward to the present, and the view of vitamin E is strikingly different. Scientific research has caught up with this remarkable nutrient. Today, with thousands of studies to support it, vitamin E is quickly being recognized as the closest thing to a "magic bullet" in the prevention of heart disease, cancer, Alzheimer's disease, and many other disorders.

So, why exactly is vitamin E so good?

Scientists tell us that age-related diseases—and the risk of most diseases increases with age—are caused in part by hazardous molecules known as free radicals. Free radicals are what makes iron rust and butter turn rancid. In a sense, they make your body more rusty and rancid with age.

Nature, however, provided a way to neutralize free radicals. The way is through a group of beneficial molecules called antioxidants. Vitamin E stands out as one of the most powerful antioxidants found in foods. It scavanges free radicals in the body and limits their damage. In doing so, vitamin E slows the aging process and reduces a person's long-term risk of age-related degenerative disease. It doesn't matter if you're a woman or a man—vitamin E can provide all people with important health benefits.

"Don't we all get enough vitamin E in the foods we eat?" you might be wondering. Over the past century, the typical American diet has undergone tremendous changes. The foods most people eat are highly processed, and vitamin E (along with many other vitamins) is removed. The typical American is consuming only a small percentage of the vitamin E his or her grandparents consumed.

In addition, our requirements for vitamin E have increased. Most people are eating more fried foods and vegetable oil than people consumed in the past. These foods are prone to causing free-radical damage in the body and increase our needs for vitamin E. Also, with increased industrialization and the increased use of polluting automobiles, people have been exposed to unprecedented levels of air pollution. Pollution also boosts our needs for vitamin E.

The question now might be "Why aren't you taking it?"

In *All About Vitamin E*, we will tell you about the remarkable story of vitamin E and how it can reduce your risk of serious degenerative diseases and even help protect you against infections. First, we will explain how vitamin E prevents heart disease, the leading cause of death among Americans and most other Westerners. Next, we'll describe the exciting research showing that vitamin E will probably reduce your long-term risk of cancer, including breast cancer in women and prostate cancer in men. Later in this book, we'll relate how vitamin E can protect you from numerous other diseases, including Alzheimer's disease and other neurological disorders, cataracts, infertility, and menopausal hot flashes. Finally, we'll explain how to shop for the best types of vitamin E.

1.

The Heart Protector

Heart disease is the leading cause of death among men and women in most Western nations. It has killed more Americans than all wars combined. Heart disease is a complex disease that develops subtly and slowly. While it has multiple causes, a lack of vitamin E is paramount among the reasons for the development of heart disease. In this chapter, we'll look at the causes of heart disease, some different aspects of this condition, and the many ways vitamin E helps prevent heart disease.

Q. Are all the claims about vitamin E being good for the heart really true?

A. Research and the clinical experiences of physicians show beyond doubt that vitamin E is good for the heart. Evidence supporting vitamin E's role as a heart protector has been building for decades. In the past several years, the evidence has become so strong that most doctors can't ignore it. For example, Harvard University researchers reported in the *New England Journal of Medicine* that vitamin E supplements dramatically reduced the risk of coronary heart disease—in both men and women. The beneficial amount used—more than 100 IU (international units)—was more than six times the Recommended Dietary Allowance (RDA) for vitamin E. This is an amount you can obtain only from supplements, not foods.

Even more impressive were the results of a blockbuster study reported in the British medical journal *Lancet*. Researchers from the University of Cambridge in England gave either 400 or 800 IU of natural vitamin E or dummy pills daily to 2,000 patients with confirmed heart disease. The group taking vitamin E for an average of eighteen months had a remarkable 77-percent lower incidence of nonfatal heart attacks than did the placebo group. The researchers pronounced vitamin E more powerful in controlling heart attacks than aspirin or cholesterol-lowering drugs—and the benefits of vitamin E were evident within only six-and-a-half months after subjects started taking it. So impressive were these results that the American Heart Association ranked vitamin E number four on its list of the top 10 heart-related popular developments in 1996.

Q. How long has it been known that vitamin E protects heart health?

A. Brace yourself for a shocking answer—it has been more than a half century since doctors first discovered that vitamin E can prevent heart disease! In the 1940s, Evan Shute, M.D., and his colleagues in London, Canada, discovered that vitamin E could reverse many symptoms of heart disease. Although their findings were described in 1946 in the respected scientific journal *Nature*, as well as in *Time* magazine, the medical establishment largely rejected their findings. Part of the reason was that most doctors at the time could not imagine how a mere vitamin would protect against the leading cause of death among Americans and Canadians. Over the years, vitamin E was ridiculed. Some people considered it a waste of money; others called it "a cure in search of a disease."

During the 1980s and 1990s, researchers quietly built a strong scientific case to support vitamin E. Simply put, vitamin E is a protective substance called an antioxidant. It neutralizes harmful substances called oxidants, or free radicals. During this time, the free-radical theory of aging—and age-related diseases—gained momentum as well. So, as an antioxidant, vitamin E could be considered an anti-aging and antidisease vitamin. The human studies conducted in the 1990s clearly demonstrated its benefits—and proved Shute was correct in his original observations that vitamin E was good for the heart.

Q. What exactly is heart disease, and how does vitamin E protect against it?

A. Heart disease (sometimes referred to as coronary artery disease) develops slowly, usually without our knowledge, in a step-by-step progression of events. It begins when artery walls become damaged or injured by free radicals. Smooth muscle cells then accumulate along artery walls, forming a plaque. Then a series of events occur that cause artery walls to become clogged with fat and cholesterol. If the artery walls become too narrow, and if the blood becomes sticky and blood clots form, blood flow can become restricted, causing a heart attack or stroke.

Vitamin E, as an antioxidant, helps protect both the artery walls and the cholesterol found in our bloodstreams from free-radical damage. Both of these mechanisms help prevent heart disease from developing and progressing.

Q. Is there any evidence vitamin E can help *reverse* heart disease?

A. Yes, there is—in both animal and human studies. Researchers have found that in monkeys, our close biological relatives, clogged arteries induced by a high-fat diet can be not only prevented but also reversed by modest amounts of vitamin E. In a six-year research project, Anthony J. Verlangieri, Ph.D., of the University of Mississippi's Atherosclerosis Research Laboratory, fed monkeys a high-fat diet that caused their arteries to become clogged and blocked. When monkeys were also given vitamin E, the extent of arterial blockage dropped 60 to 80 percent. More remarkable was the fact that arteries that were seriously clogged began to open up, from an average 35-percent artery closure to a 15-percent closure in two years!

Similarly, Howard N. Hodis, M.D., of the University of Southern California School of Medicine, Los Angeles, monitored the condition of people who had undergone bypass surgery. He found that patients taking 100 to 450 IU of vitamin E daily developed smaller lesions, or cholesterol deposits, on their arteries, compared with bypass patients not taking vitamin E supplements.

Q. What exactly are free radicals and antioxidants?

A. Free radicals are molecules with at least one unpaired electron. As a consequence, they're highly unstable and reactive, always cruising around aggressively looking for other compounds from which they can take an electron in an effort to become stabilized.

Antioxidants quench free radicals by donating electrons to make up for the missing ones in free radicals. This means that antioxidants scavenge free radicals before they cause harm to our cells. You can think of antioxidants as bodyguards that protect cells from damage by free radicals.

Free-radical damage is implicated in the development and spread of not just heart disease but all degenerative diseases, as you'll read many times throughout this book. You'll soon discover that taking antioxidants such as vitamin E is important for protecting the whole body, not just the heart, against disease.

Q. I have high cholesterol. Can vitamin E help?

A. Vitamin E won't lower high blood levels of cholesterol, but it will protect against heart disease by doing something more important—preventing the low-density lipoprotein (LDL) form of cholesterol from being chemically changed and becoming toxic to arteries.

LDL cholesterol is often referred to as the "bad" cholesterol, but it isn't really inherently bad—it is actually needed to transport vitamin E and other fat-soluble vitamins through the bloodstream. LDL, however, becomes harmful to arteries when there is insufficient vitamin E in our systems to prevent it from being oxidized or damaged by free radicals. When LDL cholesterol becomes oxidized, it infiltrates blood-vessel walls and causes fatty deposits to build up. Studies in animals and humans consistently show that 400 to 500 IU of vitamin E daily protects LDL from oxidation, thus preventing LDL deposits in blood vessels and reducing the risk of coronary heart disease.

If you take cholesterol-lowering drugs, it's especially important for you to take vitamin E. Cholesterol-lowering drugs cause vitamin E levels in LDL to drop, and LDL, in turn, oxidizes more quickly than normal. Thus, while such drugs lower cholesterol levels, they may actually increase damage to blood vessel walls.

Q. Are there other ways vitamin E helps protect against cardiovascular disease?

A. Yes, there are. Vitamin E works in a variety of ways beyond that of an antioxidant to slow or stop the development of heart disease and stroke. It slows down the buildup of smooth muscle cells on artery walls that contribute to artery-clogging plaque. In some people, vitamin E also may increase levels of the high-density lipoprotein (HDL) form of cholesterol—the type that is called the "good" cholesterol because it carries waste products from the bloodstream to the liver for elimination.

Vitamin E also decreases excessive platelet aggregation—the tendency of blood platelets to stick together and promote the formation of blood clots—which would increase the risk of heart attack and stroke. These "blood-thinning" benefits of vitamin E make it particularly important for diabetics and women who take oral contraceptives, both of whom have an increased tendency for excessive platelet aggregation and higher risk of stroke.

Q. Will vitamin E help protect my heart, even if I eat a lot of fatty foods?

The Heart Protector

A. According to recent studies, vitamin E can actually help to protect you from the effects of high-fat foods. Fatty meals normally trigger a chain of chemical reactions that tense up blood vessels. A fascinating study supervised by cardiologist Gary Plotnick, M.D., of the University of Maryland found that vitamin E and vitamin C offer significant protection against the damaging effects of high-fat meals.

In the study, twenty faculty members ate a popular high-fat fast-food breakfast consisting of eggs, sausage, muffins, and hash browns. As the researchers expected, the fat burden of this breakfast prevented the subjects' arteries from relaxing, or dilating, normally. On another day, the same subjects ate the same breakfast, but this time about fifteen minutes before the breakfast, they took 800 IU of vitamin E and 1,000 mg of vitamin C. This combination offered remarkable protection: Their blood vessels behaved normally, regularly dilating as if they had eaten low-fat foods—and the benefits lasted for six hours.

Taking these nutrient supplements in addition to choosing healthier foods offers the best protection against heart disease. However, this study shows that if you do indulge in fast food, it's smart to take vitamin E and vitamin C right before or with your meal.

Q. I'm careful to eat a healthy diet. Don't I get enough vitamin E?

A. Ironically, the answer is no. The amount of vitamin E most commonly recommended to confer benefits to the heart—400 IU—is impossible to get from foods alone. You'd have to eat 1,000 almonds or one pound of sunflower seeds—8,000 calories worth of food—to obtain this amount of vitamin E.

Vitamin E is a fat-soluble vitamin, so the best sources are foods high in fat, particularly whole wheat grains, nuts, and seeds. However, increasing your intake of fats, particularly your intake of vegetable oils, ironically boosts the need for vitamin E. The reason is that vegetable oils are prone to oxidation (free-radical damage), and extra vitamin E is needed to prevent this oxidation. So, no matter who you are or what type of diet you eat, it's necessary to take supplemental vitamin E to protect your heart.

Q. I'm about to have bypass surgery. Is it too late to start taking vitamin E?

A. No, it's never too late. But if you're scheduled for heart surgery, you should discuss taking vitamin E with your heart doctor. There is substantial research showing that vitamin E and other antioxidant vitamins can reduce the risk of complications not only from bypass surgery but from other types of surgical procedures, such as balloon angioplasty, as well.

During bypass surgery, blood flow is temporarily stopped so surgeons can graft new arteries. When the flow of oxygen-rich blood is replenished, large numbers of free radicals are generated, and these radicals can damage the heart. To protect against the free-radical damage that's common with surgery, an increasing number of heart surgeons give their patients supplements of vitamin E and other antioxidants, such as vitamin C and coenzyme Q_{10} before surgery.

Even if you've already had bypass surgery, vitamin E can still help you. Howard N. Hodis, M.D., found that bypass patients who started taking 100 to 450 IU of vitamin E developed fewer cholesterol deposits on the walls of their arteries.

Q. Why don't more doctors recommend vitamin E?

A. Years ago, doctors had no explanation for why vitamin E could prevent and effectively treat heart disease. Today, most doctors understand that vitamin E is an antioxidant that protects against heart-damaging free radicals. More and more doctors are warming up to the idea of taking vitamin E and recommending supplements to their patients.

In general, medicine has long been skeptical of the health benefits of vitamins. It has taken a long time for doctors to adjust to the idea that high doses of vitamins might be good for health. For example, it's difficult for many surgeons to recommend a nonsurgical way to treat heart disease. They have been trained as surgeons, and that's how they make their living.

Another problem has been physician education. In medical schools, doctors learn a lot about anatomy and the names of every bone in the body, but almost nothing about nutrition. The subject of nutrition is largely relegated to dietitians, who know very little about the health benefits of vitamins. After medical school, much of a physician's ongoing education is strongly influenced by the large drug companies. These companies are interested in selling expensive, proprietary drugs, not inexpensive vitamins. So drugs are what physicians hear about, not vitamins.

Q. My doctor said vitamin E is a waste of money. Is it?

A. Nobel laureate Linus Pauling, Ph.D., once said, "If a doctor isn't 'up' on something, he's 'down' on it." If your doctor tells you vitamin E is a waste of money, he or she is either uninformed, irresponsible, or behind the times in his or her medical knowledge. In a typical year, medical journals publish about 500 scientific reports on vitamin E research.

If you decide to stick with this doctor and to entrust your health to him or her, it's up to you to educate him or her—and to protect your health by taking vitamin E. Bring up the subject with your doctor in a polite, non-threatening way. You could even share this book with him or her. Even though your doctor will be skeptical about a "popular" (rather than medical) book, point him or her to the scientific references in the References section of this book. Your doctor will be able to use these references to look up everything he or she needs to know about vitamin E. If your doctor doesn't want to look up the references, and really doesn't want to have a two-way conversation with a patient, the handwriting is pretty much on the wall: this doctor is a loser—find another one.

Q. Okay, how much vitamin E should I take for my heart?

A. In general, for preventing coronary heart disease, 400 IU of natural vitamin E should be an ideal dose for most people. The natural form of vitamin E is superior to the synthetic form, and we'll explain more about the difference in Chapter 7. If you have very serious heart disease, or are taking some prescription drugs for your heart, tell your doctor of your interest in vitamin E. Sometimes people can reduce their intake of prescription drugs after they start taking vitamin E, but this is best done with your physician's guidance.

2.
The Cancer Preventer

We tend to think of cancer as a single disease, but there are more than 100 different types of cancer. They can cause different symptoms and be brought on by various factors, but virtually all develop because of damage by free radicals, the same hazardous molecules that cause heart disease. There are many preventive measures we can take to reduce our risk for cancer, and one of the most important is to take vitamin E. In this chapter, we'll look at how cancer develops, the relationship between vitamin E and cancer prevention, some of the ways vitamin E is thought to protect against specific types of cancer, and the forms of vitamin E that may be the most protective.

Q. Can vitamin E reduce my risk for cancer?

A. The scientific evidence shows that it can. In an analysis of fifty-nine human studies on vitamin and mineral supplements and cancer risk, researchers found that vitamin E supplements were the most strongly associated with a reduced cancer risk of all the supplements studied, according to an article in *Cancer Causes and Control*. Many studies have also found that high levels of vitamin E in the body are associated with a lower risk of cancer, whereas low levels are associated with a greater risk. These trends have been identified with colon cancer, lung cancer, cervical dysplasia and cancer, breast cancer, and throat cancer.

Although vitamin E can reduce the risk of cancer, do not view it as a cancer treatment (though it may be helpful with other treatments). In some studies that have found no anticancer benefits from vitamin E, the participants have smoked for years or eaten a poor diet. Smoking and an unhealthy diet are strong risk factors for cancer, so vitamin E isn't a magic bullet that can totally erase the deleterious, cumulative effects brought on by years of unhealthy living. It is, however, an essential nutrient the body needs to function properly and help ward off diseases like cancer.

Q. What is cancer, and how does it develop?

A. Cancer is a disease in which normal cell growth goes awry. It usually (but not always) develops very slowly. Most cancers begin when free radicals damage deoxyribonucleic acid (DNA, or genetic material) within your cells. DNA is a set of biological instructions that tells your cells how to function normally, so when DNA becomes damaged, the instructions that tell cells to perform properly become garbled. Even when a cell becomes cancerous, the immune system can often destroy it before it replicates and becomes established as a cancer. But when free-radical damage occurs in enough of your cells, cancerous cells can proliferate, accumulate, and spread.

Free radicals are byproducts of normal cellular processes, so they're a natural part of living. But free radicals are also generated by exposure to pollutants, radiation, and chemicals. Modern living, therefore, often tips the balance between free radicals and antioxidants (the free-radical quenchers) toward too many free radicals. Tobacco smoke tips this balance in a significant way, which is why smokers have a very high risk of most cancers (not just lung cancer). Because a big part of the process that leads to cancer involves damage from too many free radicals, the best way to protect your body against cancer is to supplement your diet with antioxidants such as vitamin E.

Q. How does vitamin E protect against cancer?

A. First and foremost, as a component of the membranes of cells, vitamin E helps prevent them from becoming damaged by free radicals from a wide variety of sources including radiation, chemicals, and toxins. Vitamin E can also prevent nitrites (certain compounds found in smoked, cured, and pickled foods) from forming nitrosamines, which are strong tumor promoters. It also may assist or accelerate the body's metabolism of carcinogenic, or cancer-causing, substances.

In addition, vitamin E appears to block the formation of blood vessels in tumors. Tumors need their own network of blood vessels in order to grow. This process of the creation of new blood vessels is a called angiogenesis. According to cell and rodent studies, vitamin E has anti-angiogenic properties. This is particularly true of the succinate form (d-alpha-tocopheryl succinate) of vitamin E. In addition, there is growing evidence that vitamin E plays a role in normal gene expression, or activation. It's very possible that vitamin E maintains normal gene activity and helps turn off abnormal gene activity characteristic of tumors.

Other research shows that cancerous tumors generate large numbers of their own free radicals, thereby creating endless mutations to circumvent various types of chemotherapeutic drugs. By quenching free radicals, vitamin E may slow down the mutation rate in cancers, enabling other treatments to fight it.

Q. Should I take other antioxidants besides vitamin E to protect against free radicals?

A. Vitamin E is recognized as the key antioxidant for protecting cellular walls against free-radical damage, so your health will certainly benefit from taking vitamin E alone. But research indicates that a diverse selection of antioxidants may be more important for protecting the body against free-radical damage than high doses of a single antioxidant. Antioxidants other than vitamin E include vitamin C, beta-carotene and other carotenoids (such as lutein and lycopene), coenzyme Q_{10}, alpha-lipoic acid, selenium, and zinc. Different antioxidants scavenge different types of free radicals, so a combination of antioxidants forms a stronger antioxidant shield to protect the body against cancer and other degenerative diseases.

Antioxidants also work synergistically with each other. Vitamin C, for example, recycles vitamin E that has been used up; selenium works in concert with vitamin E; and zinc is needed to maintain normal blood concentrations of vitamin E. Taking a combination of antioxidants, therefore, better ensures that you'll get the most mileage out of the vitamin E you take.

Q. Is there any evidence that vitamin E can reverse cancer?

A. So far there's no research to indicate that vitamin E can reverse cancer in humans. In other words, do not try to use vitamin E as a "cure" for cancer. However, one particular type of vitamin E, d-alpha tocopheryl succinate, has been found to inhibit growth of cancer cells in cell cultures (dishes of cells in a laboratory) and rodent experiments. Another group of vitamin E molecules called tocotrienols also has been found to kill human breast-cancer cells grown in cell cultures. The research so far is preliminary, but scientists are excited about the promise of both forms of vitamin E in fighting against cancer.

Although certain types of vitamin E and other nutrients may be used routinely against cancer one day, the best approach is to begin taking vitamin E to help prevent cancer. Prevention is always the best policy, especially for cancer, which can be a devastating and emotionally wrenching disease.

To put all of this a slightly different way: If either of us were diagnosed with cancer, we would take supplements of the d-alpha tocopheryl succinate form of vitamin E, in addition to pursuing other types of therapies. We would not rely on vitamin E alone, and neither should you.

Q. I'm concerned about prostate cancer. Can vitamin E protect me?

A. Vitamin E supplementation significantly lowers the risk of prostate cancer, according to recent findings in a study reported in the *Journal of the National Cancer Institute*. In the study, Ollie P. Heinonen, M.D., D.Sc., and his colleagues at the University of Helsinki tracked the health of 29,000 men for six years. The men taking vitamin E were 32-percent less likely to develop prostate cancer and 41-percent less likely to die from the disease. Beneficial effects were seen within two years of starting supplementation.

The results of this study are especially significant because the men were smokers and at above-average risk of cancer. The researchers acknowledged that the "simple intervention" of taking a vitamin E supplement may help prevent prostate cancer, which is the most frequently diagnosed cancer in men. This study used a relatively low dose—50 IU—of vitamin E, but a higher dose—400 IU—has greater overall benefits to the heart and, likely, to the prostate.

Q. Breast cancer runs in my family. Can vitamin E reduce my risk?

A. It may very well. Research with animals suggests that vitamin E can compensate to some extent for a genetic defect that increases the risk of breast cancer. To explain a bit more, some people have a genetic defect that results in low production of catalase, an antioxidant enzyme the body produces. Without sufficient catalase, cells have trouble neutralizing the free radicals that can cause breast cancer.

Japanese researchers at the Okayama University Medical School studied mice that did not produce enough catalase. They found that catalase-deficient mice were more likely than normal mice to develop breast cancer. But when the researchers added vitamin E to the mice's diet, the mice were far less likely to develop breast cancer.

Could vitamin E benefit people in the same way? According to the researchers, who published their findings in the *Japanese Journal of Cancer Research*, "Vitamin E intrinsically has a protective effect against the development of mammary tumor, and this may apply . . . to humans." Most of us won't know whether we're producing insufficient catalase or not. However, this research suggests that taking vitamin E over a lifetime may reduce the risk of breast cancer in those individuals who unknowingly produce low amounts of catalase. The benefits of vitamin E supplementation are great; the cost is relatively low.

Q. Are there other examples of vitamin E's protective effects against free-radical damage and cancer?

A. Vitamin E's ability to protect the skin from free-radical damage is one good example. The skin is regularly exposed to ultraviolet radiation from sunlight that generates large numbers of free radicals, which age the skin and greatly increase the risk of skin cancer. Skin cancer is of great concern because it is the most prevalent type of cancer, and the incidence among Americans is steadily increasing. But research in rodents has found that both internal and external use of vitamin E protects the skin from the initial damage that can occur from excessive exposure to UV radiation. It also raises levels of protective antioxidants in the skin and reduces suppression of the immune system that often occurs as a result of exposure to too much sunlight. Through these mechanisms, vitamin E makes the body better able to protect itself against skin cancer.

Another example is how vitamin E helps protect against precancerous growths in the mouth and throat. These growths are found predominantly in people who smoke tobacco or drink excessive amounts of alcohol, activities that can generate large numbers of free radicals. In a study conducted by Steven Benner, M.D., of the University of Texas Anderson Cancer Center, Houston, patients with these growths were given 400 IU of vitamin E twice daily for twenty-four weeks. About a quarter of the patients experienced a decrease of more than half in the size of their precancerous lesions, and another quarter had a complete disappearance of the growths. These are two good examples of the way vitamin E can quench free radicals from a variety of sources and thus protect against many different forms of cancer.

Q. Is there anything else I should know about vitamin E and cancer?

A. Probably the most important way vitamin E helps ward off cancer is by boosting the immune system. As mentioned earlier, cancerous cells can develop—many experts think all people have some cancer cells in their bodies—but cancerous tumors won't take hold as long as our immune systems are strong and primed to scavenge those cells. Vitamin E supplementation has been shown to boost the immune system in a variety of ways, including increasing the activity of natural killer cells. Natural killer cells are Rambo-type cells that can recognize cells that have gone bad; they're fully armed and ready to kill cancerous cells on the spot before the cells can divide and cause harm. This means that supplemental vitamin E helps keep your immune cells in a vigorous state, ready to attack the first cancer cells they see.

Q. How much vitamin E should a person take to reduce the risk of cancer?

A. As with coronary heart disease, 400 IU of natural vitamin E seems to be an effective and safe dose for cancer prevention.

3.

The Immunity Booster

Vitamin E's ability to protect against heart disease and cancer has been the focus of much research. However, its ability to boost the immune system has gone largely unnoticed until recent years. Your immune system, of course, can bolster your defenses against colds and other infections. This chapter will cover the ways vitamin E enhances immunity and how it can protect you from everything from everyday minor illnesses to more serious infections.

Q. Can vitamin E prevent me from being sick very often?

A. It should, though the effect will likely be subtle and long term instead of quick and dramatic. Several studies show that vitamin E boosts the immune system and can enhance resistance to infection. This is particularly important for older folks, because the immune system declines with age, and this causes an increased susceptibility to illness.

In one study, Simin N. Meydani, D.V.M., Ph.D., of Tufts University gave vitamin E to a group of men and women 65 years of age and older. Subjects taking 200 IUs each day for about four months showed significant improvements on various tests that assess the immune system's ability to ward off diseases. The subjects' immune responses actually behaved more like those of 40 year olds than 65 or 70 year-olds. Furthermore, the incidence of self-reported illnesses, such as colds, declined by about 30 percent. In other studies, vitamin E has been found to boost the immune responses of young people.

Q. How would a lack of vitamin E impact my health?

A. A deficiency of vitamin E can make you not only more susceptible to illness, but also more prone to virus mutations that can lead to serious disease. Generally, it's well known that nutritional deficiencies reduce the ability of the immune system to fight infections. Basically, deficiencies prevent your immune system from mounting an effective counterattack against bacteria and viruses. But there has recently been a significant development in this field.

In groundbreaking studies, Melinda Beck, Ph.D., of the University of North Carolina at Chapel Hill, and Orville Levander, Ph.D., of the U.S. Department of Agriculture, discovered that deficiencies of vitamin E or the mineral selenium in a person or animal can turn a common virus into a deadly, rapidly producing strain. Beck and Levander studied the coxsackie virus, which infects about 20 million Americans annually and usually causes no more than a sore throat, diarrhea, or coldlike symptoms. However, when a person or animal is deficient in vitamin E or selenium (a mineral that works hand in hand with vitamin E), the virus can mutate into a strain that inflames the heart muscle, leading to such heart conditions as cardiomyopathy and heart failure. Adequate levels of both nutrients, though, prevent mutations of the virus. This research provides one more convincing reason to take supplemental vitamin E (as well as selenium). Beck and Levander are currently studying how deficiencies of vitamin E and selenium might cause other viruses, such as cold and flu viruses, to mutate.

Q. How does vitamin E improve immunity?

A. The immune system mounts an amazingly complex defense against invaders, and vitamin E stimulates many parts of this defense. Specifically, vitamin E has been found to:

- Improve the function of phagocytes (cells that act as biological Pac-Men against a broad range of microorganisms).

- Stimulate activity of natural killer cells (which destroy cancer and virus-infected cells).

- Enhance the body's ability to produce antibodies (which tag or damage viruses).

- Lower levels of prostaglandin E2 (a hormonelike substance that interferes with immune function).

Through all these mechanisms, vitamin E acts as a powerful, broad-spectrum immune enhancer. And in addition to stimulating immunity, vitamin E also protects the immune system from the wear and tear of constantly defending the body from unwanted invaders. Although it's surprising to many people, immune cells like phagocytes generate enormous quantities of free radicals to kill bacteria, yet these cells are highly susceptible to damage from free radicals. Vitamin E, of course, quenches free radicals, protecting healthy cells—including immune cells—from damage.

Q. How much vitamin E should I take to protect my immunity?

A. It depends on the state of your health, but 200 to 400 IU daily would seem beneficial for most people. Higher doses of vitamin E (as well as other nutrients) may be beneficial for those with severe immunity problems.

Q. Can vitamin E help those infected with HIV?

A. Yes, it can. We'll describe some of the animal and human studies in this area. Free radicals are known to promote the replication of the HIV virus, which causes AIDS. In animal studies, vitamin E has been shown to indirectly inhibit replication of the HIV virus by quenching free radicals and by stimulating various aspects of the immune system. A number of studies have found that people infected with HIV have low levels of vitamin E and other nutrients. One recent study conducted in Toronto found that supplements of vitamins E and C reduced virus levels in people infected with HIV. All of this research suggests vitamin E may be beneficial for treating HIV infection, but more studies in humans are needed to confirm this.

It's important to recognize that people with HIV and AIDS may need far more than the standard low RDA levels of vitamins. There are many reasons for this, not the least being that many patients with AIDS suffer from diarrhea, which promotes nutrient loss. Researchers have found that patients with HIV and AIDS have low blood levels of most vitamins and minerals, and that very high supplemental amounts are usually needed to achieve "normal" blood levels of these nutrients.

Q. I have an inflammatory autoimmune condition. Will vitamin E overstimulate my immune system?

A. It's not likely to because vitamin E enhances certain types of immune cells and dampens others that are involved in inflammation. Anytime you have inflammation in the body, in fact, large numbers of free radicals accompany the inflammation, and vitamin E can serve as an antidote against these damaging molecules.

Although vitamin E boosts the immune system in many ways, it doesn't make autoimmune conditions like rheumatoid arthritis or lupus worse. To the contrary, when taken in high enough doses, vitamin E generally improves the symptoms of individuals with autoimmune conditions. In one study, for example, people with lupus receiving 900 to 1,600 IUs of vitamin E per day showed complete or almost complete clearing of symptoms; however, lower dosages of 300 IU had no effect. Patients suffering from rheumatoid arthritis have also benefited from supplementation—experiencing a lessening of pain and other common symptoms—with doses ranging from 400 to 1,200 IUs per day. Vitamin E really seems to act as a regulator or fine-tuner of the immune system.

4.

The Brain Preserver

Vitamin E is a nutrient critical for proper brain and nerve function, and supplements have been found to have beneficial effects against brain and nervous system disorders, such as Alzheimer's disease, tardive dyskinesia, and Parkinson's disease. This chapter will cover the important roles of vitamin E in brain and nerve health and how vitamin E is believed to protect against these devastating diseases.

Q. Why is vitamin E important for brain health?

A. The brain contains large amounts of polyunsaturated fatty acids (PUFAs), the types of fats most prone to free-radical damage. When the fatty acids in one brain cell become damaged, they can trigger a chain or wildfire-type reaction in which many fatty acids throughout the brain become damaged.

Vitamin E, though, can halt this wildfire reaction before it begins: it's the most important fat-soluble antioxidant to shield fatty tissues like those in the brain from damage. Taking supplemental vitamin E, therefore, helps promote optimal brain health and should lower the risk of degenerative diseases associated with free-radical damage, such as Alzheimer's disease.

Q. Is vitamin E a cure for Alzheimer's disease?

A. No, it's not a cure, but vitamin E can slow the progression of Alzheimer's disease more than a leading drug used for this purpose can. In a recent study reported in *The New England Journal of Medicine*, Mary Sano, Ph.D., of Columbia University's College of Physicians and Surgeons, New York, and her colleagues gave patients with severe Alzheimer's disease a large dose of vitamin E (2,000 IU), selegiline (a drug used to treat Parkinson's disease), a combination of them, or a placebo daily for two years. Vitamin E delayed the progression of end-stage Alzheimer's disease by almost eight months more than the placebo, which was slightly longer than the effects of selegiline. Patients taking vitamin E declined in their ability to perform daily tasks like dressing, cooking, and eating 25-percent less than did the placebo group. These kinds of abilities keep Alzheimer's disease sufferers at home rather than in a nursing home and improve quality of life. For a disease that has no known cure, these results are impressive.

Right after this study was published, the American Psychiatric Association gave its seal of approval to vitamin E, recommending it as a normal and appropriate part of the treatment of Alzheimer's disease that's safer than selegiline. Research is currently being planned to see if vitamin E will be even more effective for those with early-stage Alzheimer's disease.

Q. Why would vitamin E help protect against Alzheimer's disease?

A. Vitamin E maintains cell-membrane flexibility, and brain cells that have flexible membranes function more efficiently. Cell membranes act like the walls and doors of cells. As long as they are flexible, they allow other important nutrients into cells and waste products out. If the membranes start to get rigid, important nutrients can't get in and cellular waste products just keep accumulating inside brain cells, causing poor function and eventually destruction of brain cells, which can lead to Alzheimer's disease.

Q. Should I take vitamin E to help prevent or delay the development of Alzheimer's disease?

A. You should take vitamin E to protect health in general, and doing this should reduce your risk of developing Alzheimer's disease over the long term. It's likely that the longer you take vitamin E, the more protected against Alzheimer's disease you will be. Although the Alzheimer's study used 2,000 IU of vitamin E daily, much less is probably needed for long-term prevention. Again, an ideal preventive dose would seem to be about 400 IU daily.

Beta-amyloid is the abnormal protein that accumulates in the brains of Alzheimer's disease patients. In lab and rodent experiments, researchers have found that nerve cells die when they are exposed to beta-amyloid. But when vitamin E is added, the cells stay healthy. Many researchers in the field believe vitamin E can act preventively against Alzheimer's disease, and they take vitamin E for this reason.

If you're young, taking steps to prevent Alzheimer's disease may be the furthest thing from your mind. It shouldn't be though: Alzheimer's disease is the fourth-leading cause of death in the United States, and about five million Americans are expected to be diagnosed with it by the turn of the century.

Q. What other brain or nervous conditions can vitamin E help?

A. Vitamin E can help tardive dyskinesia, for one. This is a condition characterized by involuntary muscle movements, which often afflicts long-term alcoholics and people who have been treated with antipsychotic drugs. Like Alzheimer's disease, tardive dyskinesia is believed to be caused by free-radical damage. Several studies have found vitamin E effective in treating tardive dyskinesia, especially in patients who have had the disease for five years or less. In one scientifically controlled study of twenty-eight patients, a daily intake of 1,600 IU of vitamin E for two to three months was found to reduce involuntary muscle movements by one-third.

Q. Is vitamin E of any help in Parkinson's disease?

A. Parkinson's disease involves progressive degeneration of nerve cells in the brain, and symptoms include incapacitating tremors, rigidity, and loss of balance. There's some conflicting evidence on the effectiveness of vitamin E against Parkinson's disease, perhaps because several studies used synthetic vitamin E, which is not well absorbed into the bloodstream and used by the body. However, vitamin E still appears to be helpful. In a large-scale study of 5,342 people in the Netherlands, researchers found the risk of Parkinson's disease went up as vitamin E consumption went down.

Since free radicals are believed to be at work in Parkinson's disease, researchers at the Columbia University Department of Neurology gave high doses of vitamin E (3,200 IU), coupled with 3 grams of vitamin C, to patients with Parkinson's. The researchers found that those on the antioxidant therapy went 2.5 years longer before requiring drug therapy to treat their symptoms than those who received no antioxidants. The doctors conducting this trial concluded that "The progression of Parkinson's disease may be slowed by administration of these antioxidants."

Q. Can vitamin E enhance my memory?

A. There's no direct evidence to prove this, but vitamin E helps promote healthy brain function, and healthy brain function is needed for normal memory recall. If vitamin E is taken regularly, it's logical to think that it might help memory slightly.

In addition, brain function naturally declines as

we age, but vitamin E can slow this aging process. In an experiment involving mice, supplemental vitamin E, in amounts equivalent to a human dose of 400 IUs per day, were found to prolong the life of cells by preventing or delaying free-radical damage to a crucial strand of proteins called band-3 proteins. Some of the cells that would be most protected by vitamin E supplementation, based on this research, would be cells that perform thinking and memory functions.

Taking vitamin E is a good, long-term strategy to support brain health and keep yourself mentally sharp. If your memory has faltered some, and you're actively trying to improve it, try taking acetyl-L-carnitine and phosphatidyl serine (other nutrients that appear to be significant memory enhancers) in addition to vitamin E.

5.

The Sexual Health Vitamin for Men and Women

In the 1920s, researchers discovered that vitamin E was necessary for reproduction in rats, and people started referring to vitamin E as the sex vitamin. Although vitamin E isn't an aphrodisiac, it turns out that it does help a wide variety of reproductive problems—everything from impotence and infertility in men, to sore breasts, premenstrual syndrome, and menopausal hot flashes in women. In this chapter, we'll sort through the truths and misconceptions about vitamin E as a sex vitamin.

Q. Can vitamin E help me perform better in bed?

A. Vitamin E can help some men with impotency,

but not in the same way as the new prescription drug Viagra. Although Viagra can improve sexual performance immediately, it can be dangerous and should be avoided by those with heart or eye disease. Vitamin E works in a more subtle way to improve sexual performance and it, of course, protects heart health.

Most cases of impotence are actually related to cardiovascular disease. Basically, the blood vessels of the penis can become damaged and narrowed from a buildup of arterial plaque, just like the blood vessels that surround the heart. So anything that improves cardiovascular disease—such as vitamin E—may also help impotency. Vitamin E also improves circulation or blood flow to all tissues, including those in the penis. Every condition improves with better blood flow.

Q. My wife and I are having trouble conceiving a baby. Can vitamin E help?

A. Several studies published in *Fertility and Sterility* have reported that infertile men have low levels of antioxidants in their semen and high levels of free radicals, which can deform sperm and prevent fertilization of the egg. Vitamin E strengthens and protects the cell membranes of sperm and apparently helps them go that extra inch to father a child. In one study, Ami Amit, M.D., of Israel, gave men with normal sperm counts but low fertilization rates 200 IU of vitamin E daily for three months. The vitamin E lowered free-radical levels in the men's semen and boosted their fertilization rate by 30 percent.

It takes at least three months for vitamins to have an effect, mainly because it takes that long for sperm to mature. Infertile couples should take supplemental vitamin E and a high-potency multivitamin for several months before trying to conceive. If you smoke, try to stop because tobacco smoke inflicts free-radical damage on sperm.

Q. Can I take vitamin E if I'm pregnant?

A. Yes, you can, and you should for the health of you and your baby. Vitamin E can help protect against complications that sometimes occur during pregnancy and against those that can occur in babies that are born prematurely.

It's important, though, to ask your doctor for prenatal supplements that contain natural vitamin E instead of synthetic. Synthetic vitamin E is the type of vitamin E found in most prenatal supplements, but a recent study reported in the *American Journal of Clinical Nutrition* found that the human placenta can deliver natural vitamin E to the fetus 3.5 times more efficiently than does the synthetic supplement. Pregnancy is the most important time in life to ensure optimal nutrition, so you should give your baby and yourself the best by asking your doctor specifically for a prenatal supplement that contains natural vitamin E.

Q. My doctor told me I have fibrocystic breast disease. Can vitamin E help?

A. Fibrocystic breast disease is not a disease but a group of benign conditions affecting the breast. It usually involves lumps, cysts, and pain or tenderness in the breasts, and it's a very common condition in premenopausal women.

Several studies show that vitamin E appears to be quite effective in relieving fibrocystic breast disease symptoms, at least for many women with the condition. In one study of twenty-six women with fibrocystic breast disease, 85 percent (twenty-two women) of those who received 600 IU of vitamin E daily for eight weeks responded to treatment. In twelve women, benign cysts decreased in number and size, and in ten women, there was a total disappearance of cysts and breast tenderness.

In addition to taking vitamin E, an important strategy for alleviating fibrocystic breast disease symptoms is to strictly avoid caffeine (found in coffee, tea, cola, and chocolate). This alone can totally eradicate fibrocystic breast disease symptoms in many women.

Q. Is vitamin E of any help for PMS?

A. Vitamin E appears to work well for some women with PMS but not for everyone. Most of the research on vitamin E and premenstrual syndrome has focused primarily on breast tenderness, but at least one study suggests vitamin E may help lessen other PMS symptoms, such as nervous tension, insomnia, headache, fatigue, and depression.

Whether or not vitamin E by itself relieves premenstrual tension, you should take supplemental vitamin E as good preventive medicine to protect yourself against the leading killer of women, which is heart disease.

The best strategy to overcome PMS is a comprehensive one: Take vitamin E, but try adding supplements of B-complex vitamins, zinc, and magnesium, which have been shown to be of value. Also try avoiding all forms of sugar in your diet, which is extremely effective for alleviating PMS symptoms in many women.

Q. I've heard vitamin E eases menopausal hot flashes. Is this true?

A. Most of the research regarding this was conducted in the 1940s. Several studies found vitamin E quite effective in relieving hot flashes (as well as menopausal vaginal complaints) when compared with a dummy pill. Since then, many health-minded women have used vitamin E for these purposes, though no follow-up tests had been done.

Recently, however, researchers at the Mayo Clinic found that women can experience a reduction of hot flashes in as little as a month by taking 800 IU of supplemental vitamin E. The study was interesting because it involved 120 breast-cancer survivors who couldn't take estrogen-replacement therapy. Although estrogen-replacement therapy is the most common treatment for menopausal symptoms, such as hot flashes, it can't be used by breast-cancer survivors because it often stimulates the growth of breast cancer cells.

The breast-cancer survivors who took vitamin E experienced a small but statistically significant decrease in hot-flash activity after just four weeks, with no risk of side effects. Taking vitamin E for longer periods of time probably would provide even more beneficial effects. For women who cannot use estrogen replacement therapy—or for those who simply prefer not to—vitamin E appears to be a mild, natural substitute to ease hot flashes.

6.
The Anti-Aging Nutrient and More

Throughout this book, you've read about vitamin E's ability to prevent free-radical damage and protect against everything from heart disease to Alzheimer's disease. This chapter will cover a wide assortment of other health benefits of vitamin E—including its ability to slow the aging process, reduce the risk of cataracts, lessen exercise-induced fatigue, help heal burns, and possibly even protect against wrinkles.

Q. I've heard vitamin E called an anti-aging nutrient. Is this just hype?

A. Vitamin E is one of a number of nutrients that seem to slow the aging process. The basic idea behind this effect is that free radicals damage cells and, in effect, age them. As an antioxidant, vitamin E slows down this damage of the cells. So do other antioxidants, such as vitamin C and coenzyme Q_{10}. Since your body is essentially composed of around 100 billion cells, slowing the aging process of these individual cells will slow the aging of your entire body.

Another way to look at vitamin E's effects on aging is in terms of its effects in reducing your risk of some of the top disease killers, such as heart disease, cancer, and Alzheimer's disease. Scientific studies have shown pretty clearly that vitamin E reduces the risk of developing these diseases. It might not completely eliminate the risk—but for the sake of discussion, let's assume that vitamin E only delays the onset of these diseases. This means that you might not develop heart disease until you're 80 years old, instead of 60. If vitamin E delays the onset of these serious diseases by ten, twenty, or thirty years, you're going to live longer.

Realistically, then, vitamin E can slow the aging process—that is, the speed at which your body's cells age. It is not an "anti-aging" vitamin in the strict sense, because aging is an inevitable process. Vitamin E will not turn a 40-year-old man into a teenager. It may, however, help restore the heart function of a 70-year-old to that of someone ten or twenty years younger. But remember, eating a good diet, exercising, and minimizing stresses in your life also retard the aging process.

Q. Can vitamin E help protect my vision as I get older?

A. Vitamin E supplementation significantly reduces the risk of cataracts, which account for 42 percent of all vision loss. Cataracts are considered an age-related disorder and the leading cause of blindness worldwide.

Free radicals from pollution and ultraviolet radiation damage the proteins that form the lens of the eye and cause cataracts, so it isn't surprising that vitamin E can delay the onset and slow the progression of cataracts. In a recent study among 744 senior citizens, those who took vitamin E supplements had a 57-percent lower risk of developing cataracts.

Q. Would vitamin E be of help in treating diabetes?

A. Vitamin E should reduce the risk of many complications of diabetes, including premature aging and accelerated heart disease. High levels of glucose (blood sugar) are the chief characteristic of diabetes. Part of the disease process results from free radicals spinning off from these high glucose levels. So anything you can do to reduce free radicals should ease some of the complications of diabetes.

While vitamin E is extremely safe, some caution is required in diabetes. If you are taking insulin or hypoglycemic drugs, you may have to reduce the dosage of these drugs. This is because vitamin E will improve your health and the function of your body's insulin, so that you will need less of these drugs. However, it is very important that you adjust the dosage of vitamin E and the drugs in cooperation with your physician.

In addition, people with "leaky" blood vessels, such as in some types of diabetic retinopathy (eye disease), could develop problems with vitamin E supplements. This is because vitamin E is a mild anticoagulant. While such problems are not common, caution is warranted.

Q. Can vitamin E prevent wrinkles?

A. Wrinkles are an age-related condition that develops over time, just like heart disease and Alzheimer's disease. Vitamin E slows down the aging process, so it probably can help delay the appearance of wrinkles, especially when used as part of a comprehensive program to maintain youthful skin.

Many factors contribute to the formation and deepening of wrinkles, including poor nutrition, exposure to environmental pollutants, smoking, and especially too much time in the sun. The damaging effects of sunlight on the skin are cumulative, but they may not be obvious until years later. The best approach to preventing wrinkles is to eat well, avoid exposure to cigarette smoke and pollutants, limit your time in the sun, and take antioxidants such as vitamin E and vitamin C that help protect against the damage from sunlight, which ages the skin.

Q. I've heard vitamin E can act as a sunscreen. Is there any truth to this?

A. A recent study in the *Journal of the American Academy of Dermatology* found that taking vitamins C and E can help protect against sunburn. It does this not by acting as a sunscreen, but by enhancing the body's ability to withstand burning.

In the study, Bernadette Eberlein-Konig, M.D., and her colleagues from the dermatology clinic at the Technical University of Munich exposed twenty men and women to ultraviolet (UV) light. Then Eberlein-Konig gave half of the subjects either a placebo or supplements containing 2,000 mg of vitamin C and 1,000 IU of natural vitamin E daily for eight days, and portions of the subjects' skin were again exposed to UV light. People taking vitamin C and E showed an increased resistance to sunburn, while those taking the placebo showed an increased sensitivity to UV light.

"This study shows for the first time that systemic administration of vitamins C and E reduces the sunburn reaction in humans . . . Systemic photoprotection is convenient and could provide a desirable basic UV shield for the entire body surface," Eberlein-Konig wrote in the study.

Previous research has shown that topical applications of vitamins C and E have a weak sun-blocking effect, so using vitamin E internally and externally (both as an oral supplement and as an ingredient in topical lotions) appears to be the best way to protect yourself from damaging UV rays when you do spend time in the sun.

Q. Is there any advantage to putting vitamin E on burns and cuts?

A. Minor burns are a lot like sunburns. In burns and cuts, free radicals flood the site of injury, causing inflammation and redness. These free radicals are supposed to prevent infection, but sometimes the body doesn't know when to turn them off. An ointment containing vitamin E should help the healing process and restore normal vitamin E levels in the skin. You can also pierce vitamin E capsules with a needle and apply the oil to any minor household burns and cuts after a scab has formed.

More severe burns generate very large quantities of free radicals, which can slow the healing process. Vitamin E can quench many of these free radicals. However, the problem is more pragmatic: how do you apply vitamin E to a serious burn, when the burned person is likely to scream in pain? One company (Carlson Laboratories, 1-800-323-4141) sells a vitamin E spray that can be helpful in such cases.

Evan Shute, M.D., who pioneered the clinical use of vitamin E in heart disease, believed that his lasting contribution to medicine would be the use of vitamin E in treating burns. Shute treated many burn victims with vitamin E. It consistently promoted healing and minimized scarring.

Q. Sometimes, when I exercise, I really feel wiped out. Can vitamin E help?

A. Aerobic activity, including running, walking, bicycling, and cross-country skiing, increases the production of free radicals, which can damage muscle tissue and result in inflammation and aching muscles. But vitamin E acts like a sponge, soaking up those free radicals before they damage tissues. In a study by German researchers, regular exercise increased levels of DNA damage in human subjects. However, when the subjects took vitamin E supplements, exercise-induced DNA damage was virtually eliminated.

According to Lester Packer, Ph.D., a researcher at the University of California, Berkeley, and one of the foremost authorities on antioxidants, vitamin E can probably reduce exercise-induced fatigue. Quicker recovery from fatigue should in turn improve exercise performance.

Q. Can vitamin E protect me against secondhand cigarette smoke?

A. It can. Cigarette smoke, like other forms of air pollution, increase a person's free-radical burden. Even if you don't smoke, it could be a problem. Nonsmoking spouses of smokers are 3.5 times more likely to develop lung cancer than people living in smoke-free houses. Breathing cigarette smoke passively is comparable to smoking anywhere from one to ten cigarettes yourself daily.

When a nonsmoker breathes in smoke from a spouse, friend, or coworker, the many pollutants and cancer-causing chemicals in tobacco smoke attack the membranes and DNA of his or her body's cells. If you live with or work with a smoker, you are, in effect, a smoker. Vitamin E can help reduce the damage, as can opening the window.

Q. What else does vitamin E do?

A. Vitamin E protects lung function. In a study of 178 men and women, it was found that those who consumed the most vitamin E had significantly better lung function than those who consumed the least amount.

Vitamin E also protects red blood cells from damage. Without enough vitamin E, red blood cells die sooner than they should. Adequate vitamin E, therefore, is needed to prevent hemolytic anemia and the lethargy and depression that usually accompany this condition.

Q. Vitamin E sounds almost too good to be true. Is it a panacea?

A. A panacea is a cure-all, and vitamin E isn't quite that. However, it plays numerous roles in health, so it is not entirely surprising that vitamin E benefits a wide range of different conditions. Vitamin E is required by every cell in the body, which is why it benefits cells as different as heart and brain cells. It also plays roles in the behavior of genes, and genes contain the most basic biological instructions for the body. When Drs. Evan and Wilfrid Shute were using vitamin E in the 1940s and

1950s, many of their critics also said that vitamin E seemed like a panacea. What they were lacking was an explanation of why vitamin E works. Today, we have that explanation, and time has largely proved the Shutes right about vitamin E and its many benefits.

7.

Buying and Taking Your Vitamin E Supplement

By now, you should be convinced of the health benefits provided by vitamin E. One of the best things you could do for your health is to begin taking vitamin E supplements. While doing so might seem as simple as buying a bottle of vitamin E, finding a quality product can often be difficult and confusing. In this chapter, we explain the important differences between natural and synthetic vitamin E and the many different forms of this vitamin. We also offer a number of tips to help you choose among the many different types of vitamin E supplements.

Q. What exactly is vitamin E?

A. Vitamin E is an essential nutrient. It is a fat-soluble vitamin (in contrast to water-soluble nutrients, such as vitamin C), which means that it functions primarily in the fatty portions of cells. It also means that vitamin E supplements are best taken with a little fat or oil (such as in a regular meal) for optimal absorption. The Recommended Dietary Allowance is 15 IU daily for an adult. Unfortunately, the average American gets only about 8 IU from the diet. Furthermore, vitamin E requirements increase with higher intake of polyunsatured fatty acids (PUFAs)—the types of fats used in fried foods and salad dressings. Americans generally eat so many PUFAs that they need to compensate for the damaging effects of these fats.

Q. Vegetable oils are a good source of vitamin E, aren't they?

A. Vegetables oils are rich in PUFAs, and a person's vitamin E requirements increase when he or she consumes a lot of PUFAs. The vitamin E is needed to prevent PUFAs from oxidizing, or turning rancid. For example, a person eating fried chicken and French fries several times a week is consuming a huge quantity of PUFAs. This person is going to need a lot more vitamin E than would a vegetarian not eating any fried foods at all.

There's also a common misconception that common vegetable oils, such as soybean or peanut oil, are good dietary sources of vitamin E. Such oils tend to be very high in the gamma-tocopherol, not alpha-tocopherol, form of vitamin E. (Tocopherol is the chemical term to describe vitamin E, and the alpha fraction of the vitamin E molecule is the most active in the human body.) Although gamma-tocopherol has some antioxidant properties, the body needs primarily the alpha-tocopherol form of vitamin E. It's possible that the consuming of a lot of vegetable oils also interferes with the body's use of alpha-tocopherol.

Q. What's the most important thing to know when shopping for vitamin E?

A. The most important thing to know is that natural forms of vitamin E are far better than synthetic forms. For years, researchers believed that natural vitamin E was 1.36 times more potent than synthetic vitamin E when measured in milligrams (mg). This was a difference found in animal studies. Because of this difference, the international unit (IU) standard was developed. This way, one international unit of synthetic vitamin E is equivalent to one international unit of natural vitamin E. However, there are still major differences between natural and synthetic.

In recent human studies, Graham Burton, Ph.D.,

and Robert Acuff, Ph.D., found that natural vitamin E was absorbed and retained twice as well as synthetic vitamin E. Basically, when people were given equal amounts of natural and synthetic vitamin E, levels of natural vitamin E rose twice as high in the bloodstream and in tissues. The reason, according to a number of researchers, is that the human body selects for the natural molecule over synthetic replicas. This means that, even using the IU standard, natural vitamin E is better absorbed—and that the synthetic falls way short. Buying natural vitamin E, therefore, gives you much more value for your money.

Q. How can I distinguish between natural and synthetic vitamin E?

A. It's easy, but you have to read the fine print on the label. Natural vitamin E is identified as *d-alpha* tocopherol, whereas the synthetic is *dl-alpha* tocopherol. Natural vitamin E will be more expensive than the synthetic, but then you get what you pay for.

Q. What are the different types of natural vitamin E?

A. There are several different types. One is called *d-alpha tocopherol*. This is a natural and highly absorbable form of vitamin E. The only drawback to it is a relatively limited shelf life, though it is stable for at least three years, provided it is stored in a cool, dry environment.

Another natural form of vitamin E, *d-alpha tocopheryl acetate,* is more stable in terms of shelf life. The acetate means it has been esterified—essentially combined with a molecule similar to vinegar—to improve stability and shelf life. This is probably the best form for people actively trying to prevent heart disease, because it has been used in many medical studies.

Still another natural form of vitamin E, *d-alpha tocopheryl succinate,* which we discussed in Chapter 2, is another stable form of vitamin E. The most promising studies on vitamin E's anticancer properties have used this particular form.

Perhaps the most "nature-like" form of vitamin E is *mixed natural tocopherols*. This type of product contains a specific amount of natural d-alpha tocopherol, plus natural beta-, gamma-, and delta-tocopherols. Although alpha-tocopherol is the most biologically active form of vitamin E, the other fractions also have antioxidant properties and are believed to be of benefit.

Bear in mind that the natural d-alpha form is the most biologically active. In contrast, the synthetic vitamin E contains only about 12 percent of this form.

Q. Which type of vitamin E is best to take?

A. The answer to that question varies according to the individual. Each of the natural forms of vitamin E is good, though they have slightly different properties. After understanding the merits and drawbacks of each type (explained in the previous answer), you should evaluate which type is best for you based on what diseases you're most at risk for and what you eat.

It's important to know that all four types of tocopherols are found in natural foods, but d-alpha tocopherol is the one that's stripped away the most in processed foods (such as commercial vegetable oils and refined pasta and baked goods). If you eat a lot of processed foods, supplementing your diet with d-alpha tocopherol may be a way to compensate for some of what you're missing in your diet.

However, if you eat a lot of unprocessed, nutrient-dense, natural foods (which you should strive to do for better health), a mixed natural tocopherol supplement is probably a better choice because it more closely reproduces the way vitamin E occurs in nature, with all four tocopherols. For disease prevention, our personal preference is a mixed natural tocopherol vitamin E supplement.

Q. What's the best dose?

A. In general, most adults would do well taking 400 IU daily of natural vitamin E. This dosage reduces the oxidation of cholesterol and, based on human studies, leads to dramatic reductions in the incidence of coronary heart disease. Higher doses can further reduce the oxidation of cholesterol, but it might be better to take a combination of antioxidants than to take very high doses of vitamin E.

Antioxidants work as a team of synergistic nutrients. So as good as vitamin E is, a combination of antioxidants is preferable. Consider taking 400 IU of vitamin E, 1,000 mg or more of vitamin C, 15,000 to 25,000 mg of mixed carotenoids, 30 mg of coenzyme Q_{10}, and 50 mg of alpha-lipoic acid. Many antioxidant formulas contain these and other antioxidants and enable you to simplify the number of tablets or capsules you take.

Q. Is taking wheat germ oil just as good as taking vitamin E supplements?

A. Wheat germ oil is an excellent source of vitamin E, but it doesn't provide as much vitamin E as a small tablet or capsule. Some people also have sensitivities to wheat germ oil. Most natural vitamin E supplements, by the way, are produced from soybeans.

Q. Is there anyone who shouldn't take vitamin E?

A. Every adult should probably be taking vitamin E supplements. People who live in very polluted cities or those who exercise strenuously, live in high altitudes, or eat large amounts of fried foods or vegetable oils should probably take at least 400 IU daily, even if they are currently healthy. Children should also take vitamin E, but the dosage should be adjusted according to their weight.

Q. How safe is vitamin E?

A. Vitamin E is exceptionally safe. Clinical trials of vitamin E supplementation at doses as high as 3,200 IU daily in a wide variety of people for up to two years have not shown any unfavorable side effects.

There are some risks you should be aware of though. Although vitamin E reduces the risk of heart disease and thrombotic stroke (caused by blood clots), it slightly increases the risk of hemorrhagic stroke (caused by leaky blood vessels). The risk, in general, is insignificant because the vast majority of strokes are caused by blood clots, which vitamin E can help prevent.

Along this line, some research has shown that vitamin E supplements might amplify the effects of prescription anticoagulant (or blood-thinning) drugs. However, some research has also shown that vitamin E does not have this effect. We suspect that the effect may be dose related. If you're taking aspirin *and* a prescription anticoagulant *and* vitamin E, the combined anticoagulant effect may be a bit too much. If you are taking an anticoagulant drug, discuss your desire to take vitamin E with your physician.

Diabetics may have to adjust their dosage of insulin or hypoglycemic drugs when taking vitamin E—this is a good sign, because it indicates that their diabetic symptoms are lessening. And people with rheumatic heart disease, in which half the heart is damaged, should start taking only 50 to 100 IU of vitamin E under a physician's supervision. The reason is that the stronger part of the heart may respond much faster than the weaker part to vitamin E.

Q. What are tocotrienols? Should I get a vitamin E supplement that contains them?

A. Tocotrienols are related to tocopherols (vitamin E) but they have small differences in structure. Like tocopherols, tocotrienols have antioxidant activity. Natural sources of tocotrienols, such as palm and rice bran oil, always contain a mixture of tocotrienols and tocopherols.

Research into the benefits of tocotrienols is just beginning. One study in humans suggests tocotrienol supplements may decrease the amount of cholesterol-laden plaque in the carotid artery, the main artery that supplies blood to the brain. This would be of benefit to people prone to strokes. Other research shows tocotrienols can inhibit the growth of cancer cells grown in cell cultures.

As more becomes known about tocotrienols, we'll all learn more about exactly who would benefit from tocotrienol supplementation. Based on the research to date, those prone to stroke or cancer may want to discuss adding tocotrienols to a complete supplement program for these conditions with their doctor. It's important to understand, though, that tocotrienols do not function in exactly the same way as tocopherols. If you decide to take tocotrienol supplements for their antioxidant benefits, you should take them in addition to a tocopherol form of vitamin E.

Q. How do I know if vitamin E is working?

A. Occasionally people will experience quick relief from something like sore breasts by taking vitamin E—or they'll see evidence of cuts and burns healing faster. But most often vitamin E just works subtly and preventively, helping to slow the aging process and prevent degenerative diseases. On a day-to-day basis, you probably won't notice that your body has fewer damaging free radicals, but your risk of disease will lessen over the long term because of this benefit. The longer you take vitamin E, the more you'll probably find that you're in better health than other people your age who don't take vitamin E.

Q. Does optimal intake of vitamin E ensure good health?

A. Taking vitamin E supplements can significantly lower your risk of heart disease, enhance the functioning of your immune system, and likely reduce your risk of developing Alzheimer's disease.

Vitamin E, however, is not a magic bullet or panacea. You can't simply take a pill and expect to gain perfect health. The other components of health include eating a diet rich in fruits and vegetables, exercising moderately (at least going for a walk several times a week), and managing psychological stresses. Vitamin E supplements, in combination with a general antioxidant formula or multivitamin, can provide many health benefits—and increase your likelihood of having a long, functional, and satisfying life.

Conclusion

Vitamin E is the main antioxidant that protects all cells from damage, so it's one of the most important nutrient supplements you can take to keep your whole body healthy and protected against disease. As you've learned, vitamin E helps protect against leading killers, such as heart disease, cancer, and Alzheimer's disease. It enhances the immune system, bolstering the body's defenses against colds and other infections. Vitamin E also slows the aging process, probably delaying the onset of conditions such as cataracts and wrinkles. And it helps heal or alleviate many minor health complaints—including everything from burns to menopausal hot flashes.

If you didn't pay much attention to vitamin E until reading this book, you're probably amazed at just how much of a health protector vitamin E really is. Research on the many benefits of vitamin E continues to pile up at a furious pace, and these benefits impress virtually everyone, from once-skeptical doctors to questioning health reporters. To tap the potential of all vitamin E's benefits, though, you must take supplements of the nutrient. You simply can't get enough vitamin E for therapeutic effects from foods alone.

Numerous supplements receive a lot of hype these days, and many deliver on their promises. Vitamin E, though, is one that has stood the test of time in both scientific research and clinical practice. It's a tried-and-true nutrient supplement that should be a part of everyone's supplement regimen for better health.

In sum, do as we do: weigh the evidence, and take vitamin E supplements.

Glossary

Antioxidant. A substance, such as vitamin E, that limits damage from free radicals by donating an electron. Antioxidant nutrients can reduce the risk of heart disease and cancer. *See also* Free radical.

D-alpha tocopherol. The type of vitamin E regarded as the standard because it has the most biological activity.

Fat-soluble vitamin. A vitamin that dissolves only in oil and is found in the fatty parts of food. To be absorbed best, fat-soluble vitamins like vitamin E should be consumed with a small amount of fat.

Free radical. A molecule with an unpaired electron produced by the body and by pollutants. Free radicals are regarded as an underlying cause of aging, heart disease, and cancer. *See also* Antioxidant.

International unit (IU). An internationally standardized unit of weight, usually used for fat-soluble vitamins.

Mixed tocopherols. A term used to describe the collection of all the tocopherols in vitamin E that occur naturally in food. There are four types of tocopherols: d-alpha, d-beta, d-gamma, and d-delta tocopherols.

Polyunsaturated fatty acids (PUFAs). The types of fat found in corn, soybean, safflower, and sunflower oils that are most prone to free-radical damage. The higher your intake of PUFAs the more your need for vitamin E increases.

Tocotrienols. A group of vitamin E compounds that differ slightly from tocopherols but also have antioxidant properties. There are four types of tocotrienols: d-alpha, d-beta, d-gamma, and d-delta tocotrienols.

Vitamin. A micronutrient essential for life and health that must be obtained from food or supplements.

Vitamin E. The body's principal fat-soluble antioxidant that is incorporated into cell membranes and protects cells throughout the body from free-radical damage. There are two classes of vitamin E—tocopherols and tocotrienols.

References

The information in this book is drawn from several hundred scientific references. These are some of those references.

Burton GW, Traber MG, Acuff RV, et al., "Human plasma and tissue a-tocopherol concentrations in response to supplementation with deuterated natural and synthetic vitamin E," *American Journal of Clinical Nutrition* 67 (1998):669–684.

Eberlein-König B, Placzek M, Pryzybilla B, "Protective effect against sunburn of combined systemic ascorbic acid (vitamin C) and d-a-tocopherol (vitamin E)," *Journal of the American Academy of Dermatology* 38 (1998):45–48.

Heinonen OP, Albanes D, Virtano J, et al., "Prostate cancer and supplementation with a-tocopherol; and b-carotene: incidence and mortality in a controlled trial," *Journal of the National Cancer Institute* 90 (1998):440–446.

Ishi, K, et al., "Prevention of mammary tumorigenesis in acatalasemic mice by vitamin E supplementation," *Japanese Journal of Cancer Research* 87 (1996):680–684.

Kodama H, Yamaguchi R, Fukuda J, et al., "Increased oxidative deoxyribonucleic acid damage in the spermatozoa of infertile male patients," *Fertility and Sterility* 68 (1997):519–524.

Meydani, S, Meydani, M, et al., "Vitamin E supplementation and in vivo immune response in healthy elderly subjects," *Journal of the American Medical Association* 27 (1997):1380–1386.

Packer L, "Oxidants, antioxidant nutrients and the athlete," *Journal of Sports Sciences* 15 (1997):353–363.

Plotnick GD, Corretti MC, Vogel RA, "Effect of antioxidant vitamins on the transient impairment of endothelium-dependent brachial artery vasoactivity following a single high-fat meal," *Journal of the American Medical Association* 278 (1997):1682–1686.

Poulin, JE, Cover, C, Gustafson MR, Kay, MB, "Vitamin E prevents oxidative modification of brain and lymphocyte band 3 proteins during aging,"

Proceedings of the National Academy of Sciences 93 (1996):5600–5603.

Rimm, EB, et al., "Vitamin E consumption and the risk of coronary heart disease in men," *New England Journal of Medicine* 328 (1993):1450–1456.

Sano, M, Ernesto, C, Thomas, RG, et al, "A controlled trial of selegiline, alpha-tocopherol, or both as treatment for Alzheimer's disease," *The New England Journal of Medicine* 336 (1997):1216–1222.

Stampfer, MJ, et al., "Vitamin E consumption and the risk of coronary heart disease in women," *New England Journal of Medicine* 328 (1993):1444–1449.

Stephens NG, Parsons A, Schofield PM, et al., "Randomised controlled trial of vitamin E in patients with coronary disease: Cambridge Heart Antioxidant Study (CHAOS)," *Lancet* 347 (1996): 781–786.

Verlangieri, A. "Effects of a-tocopherol supplementation on experimentally induced primate atherosclerosis," *Journal of American College of Nutrition* 11(2) (1992):130–137.

Suggested Readings and Resources

Literature

Balch JF and Balch PA. *Prescription for Nutritional Healing*, second edition. Garden City Park, NY: Avery Publishing Group, 1997.

———. *Prescription for Nutritional Healing A-to-Z Guide to Supplements*. Garden City Park, NY: Avery Publishing Group, 1998.

Challem J. *All About Vitamins*. Garden City Park, NY: Avery Publishing Group, 1998.

Challem J and Dolby V. *Homocysteine: The Secret Killer*. New Canaan, CT: Keats, 1997.

Huemer RP and Challem J. *The Natural Health Guide to Beating the Supergerms*. New York: Pocket Books, 1997.

Lieberman S and Bruning N. *The Real Vitamin and Mineral Book* Garden City Park, NY: Avery Publishing Group, 1997.

Web (Internet) Sites
Medline (for specific medical journal abstracts):
   http://www.nlm.nih.gov/databases/freemedl.html

The Nutrition Reporter (for summaries of research):
   http://www.nutritionreporter.com

VERIS Research Information Service (for abstracts of antioxidant research):
   http://www.veris-online.org

Index

Acuff, Robert, 70
Aging and vitamin E, 57–58, 60–61
Alpha-lipoic acid, 27
Alzheimer's disease and vitamin E, 44–47
American Heart Association, 10
American Journal of Clinical Nutrition, 53
American Psychiatric Association, 45
Amit, Ami, 53
Anemia, hemolytic, 65
Antioxidants, 11–12, 14, 19, 25, 27–28, 31, 39, 73
 types of, 27–28
Autoimmune conditions and vitamin E, 40–41

Beck, Melinda, 37

Benner, Steven, 32
Beta-amyloid, 46
Beta-carotene, 27
Brain function, 43–49
 Alzheimer's disease, 44–47
 memory enhancement, 48–49
 Parkinson's disease, 47–48
 tardive dyskinesia, 47
 vitamin E and, 43–44
Breast cancer and vitamin E, 30–31
Burns, 62–63
Burton, Graham, 69–70
Bypass surgery, 18–19

Cancer, 23–33
 breast cancer, 30–31
 causes of, 24–25
 prostate cancer, 29–30

skin cancer, 31–32
vitamin E and, 23–24, 26–27, 28–29, 31–32
vitamin E dosage for, 33
Cancer Causes and Control, 24
Cardiovascular disease. *See* Heart disease.
Catalase, 30–31
Cataracts and vitamin E, 59
Cholesterol levels, high, 14–15
Coenzyme Q_{10}, 27
Coronary artery disease. *See* Heart disease.
Coxsackie virus, 37
Cuts and vitamin E, 62–63

D-alpha tocopherol, 70, 71–72
D-alpha tocopheryl acetate, 71
D-alpha tocopheryl succinate, 28, 71
Deoxyribonucleic acid (DNA), 25
Diabetes and vitamin E, 59–60
Dl-alpha tocopherol, 70

DNA. *See* Deoxyribonucleic acid.

Eberlein-Konig, Bernadette, 61
Exercise fatigue and vitamin E, 63–64

Fatty foods and vitamin E, 16–17
Fertility and Sterility, 52
Fibrocystic breast disease and vitamin E, 54–55
Free radicals
aging and, 57–59, 60–61
brain function and, 44, 47, 48, 49
burns and, 62–63
cancer and, 25, 26–27, 31–32
cuts and, 62
described, 11, 14
heart disease and, 12, 15, 19
HIV and, 39
inflammation and, 40, 63–64
sources of, 64

Glucose, 59

HDL. *See* High-density-lipoprotein cholesterol.
Heart attack. *See* Heart disease.
Heart disease, 9–22
  causes of, 12
  prevention of, 9–12, 14–17
  reversal of, 13
  vitamin E dosage for, 21–22
Heinonen, Ollie P., 29
Hemolytic anemia, 65
Hemorrhagic stroke, 75
High-density-lipoprotein (HDL) cholesterol, 16
High-fat foods and vitamin E, 16–17
HIV and vitamin E, 39–40
Hodis, Howard N., 13, 19
Hot flashes and vitamin E, 55–56

Immunity, 35–41
  effects of vitamin E on, 32–33, 37–41
  vitamin-E deficiency and, 36–37
  vitamin E dosage for, 39

Impotence and vitamin E, 52
Infertility and vitamin E, 52–53
Inflammation and vitamin E, 40–41

Japanese Journal of Cancer Research, 30
Journal of the American Academy of Dermatology, 61
Journal of the National Cancer Institute, 29

Lancet, 10
LDL. *See* Low-density-lipoprotein cholesterol.
Levander, Orville
Low-density-lipoprotein (LDL) cholesterol, 15
Lung function and vitamin E, 65
Lutein, 27
Lycopene, 27

Mayo Clinic, 56
Memory enhancement and vitamin E, 48–49
Meydani, Simin N., 36

Mixed natural tocopherols, 71, 72

Nature, 11
New England Journal of Medicine, 10, 44

Oxidants. *See* Free radicals.

Packer, Lester, 64
Parkinson's disease, 47–48
Phagocytes, 38
Platelet aggregation, 16
Plotnik, Gary, 17
PMS. *See* Premenstrual syndrome.
Polyunsaturated fatty acids (PUFAs), 43–44, 68–69
Pregnancy, 53–54
Premenstrual syndrome (PMS), 55
Prostaglandin E2, 38
Prostate cancer and vitamin E, 29–30

Recommended Dietary Allowance (RDA) for vitamin E, 10, 68
Secondhand smoke, 64
Selegiline, 44–45
Selenium, 27, 37
Sexual health, 51–56
 fibrocystic breast disease, 54–55
 hot flashes, 55–56
 impotence, 51–52
 infertility, 52–53
 pregnancy, 53–54
 premenstrual syndrome (PMS), 55
Shute, Evan, 11, 65–66
Shute, Wilfrid, 65–66
Skin cancer and vitamin E, 31–32
Sunburn, prevention of, 61–62

Tardive dyskinesia and vitamin E, 47
Time, 11
Tocopherols, 70–71, 76–77
Tocotrienols, 76–77

Vegetable oils, vitamin E in, 68–69
Verlangieri, Anthony J., 13
Viagra, 52
Vision and vitamin E, 59
Vitamin C, 17, 27
Vitamin E

and aging, 57–58, 60–61
and Alzheimer's disease, 44–47
as an antioxidant, 11–12, 14, 19, 25, 26–27, 31–32, 39, 77
and autoimmune conditions, 40–41
and brain function, 43–49
and breast cancer, 30–31
and cancer, 23–33
and cataracts, 59
and cuts, 62–63
and diabetes, 59–60
doctor recommendation of, 19–21
and exercise fatigue, 63–64
and fibrocystic breast disease, 54–55
function of, 11–12, 67–68
and heart disease, 9–13, 14–15, 16
and HIV, 39–40
and hot flashes, 55–56
and immunity, 32–33, 37–38
and infertility, 52–53
and inflammation, 40–41
and lung function, 65
and memory enhancement, 48–49
and prostate cancer, 29–30
safety of, 74–75
and sexual health, 51–56
and skin cancer, 31–32
sources of, 18, 68–69
suggested dosage for, 74
and vision, 59
and wrinkles, 60–61
Vitamin-E deficiency, effects of, 36–37
Vitamin-E supplements
buying, 69–70
natural, 53–54, 70–72
suggested dosage, 73
synthetic, 53–54, 70

Wheat germ oil, 73–74
Wrinkles and vitamin E, 60–61

Zinc, 27